GUT HEALTH COOKBOOK

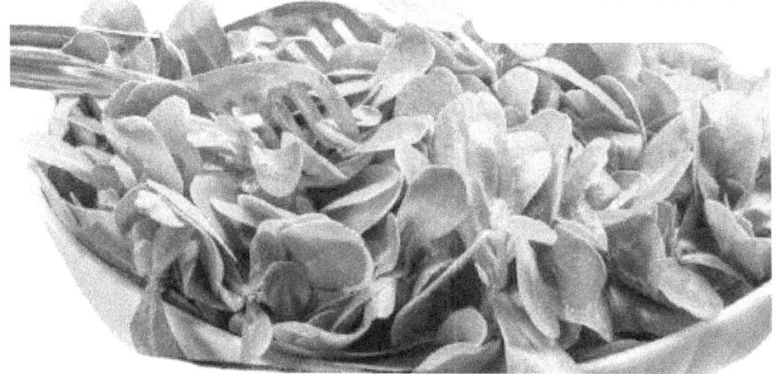

DR. JESSICA SMITH

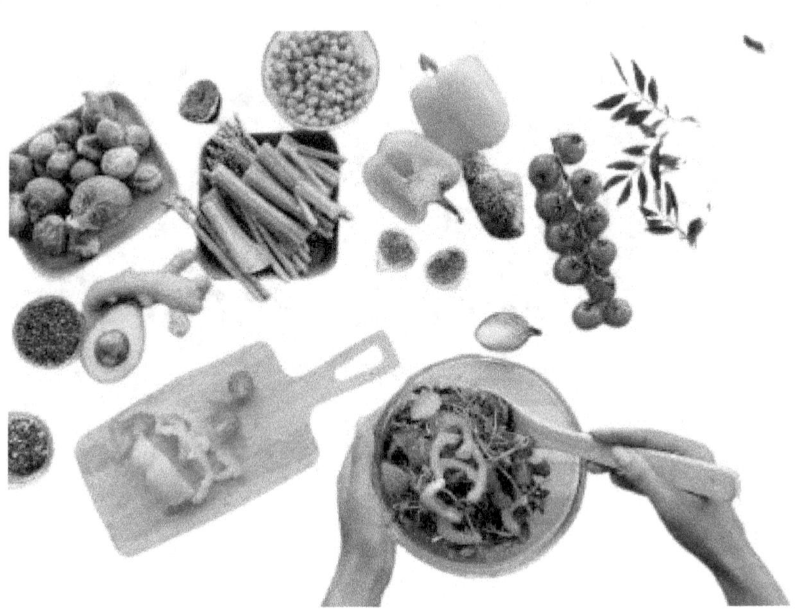

TABLE OF CONTENT

HOW TO USE A GUT HEALTH COOKBOOK

Using a gut health cookbook can be a beneficial and delicious way to support your digestive system. Here's a general guide on how to make the most of a gut health cookbook:

Select a Cookbook:

Choose a cookbook that focuses on gut-friendly recipes. Look for titles that mention "gut health," "digestive wellness," or "gut-friendly meals."

Understand the Basics of Gut Health:

Familiarize yourself with the fundamentals of gut health. Understand the importance of probiotics, prebiotics, fiber, and fermented foods in supporting a healthy gut microbiome.

Read the Introduction:

Most gut health cookbooks provide an introduction that discusses the importance of gut health and may include tips on how to incorporate gut-friendly ingredients into your diet.

Check for Guidelines:

Look for any specific guidelines or recommendations provided by the author. This could include information on portion sizes, meal frequency, or dietary restrictions.

Stock Up on Gut-Friendly Ingredients:

Ensure your kitchen is stocked with gut-friendly ingredients such as:

Probiotic-rich foods (yogurt, kefir, sauerkraut, kimchi)

Prebiotic-rich foods (garlic, onions, leeks, bananas, asparagus)

High-fiber foods (whole grains, fruits, vegetables, legumes)

Fermented foods (kombucha, miso, tempeh)

Follow Recipes Carefully:

Pay close attention to the recipes in the cookbook. Follow the instructions, including measurements and cooking times, to ensure you're preparing the meals correctly.

Experiment with New Ingredients:

Embrace the opportunity to try new ingredients that are beneficial for gut health. Don't be afraid to experiment with different grains, vegetables, and fermented products.

Include a variety of Foods:

Ensure that your meals include a variety of nutrient-dense foods. Incorporate a mix of colors, textures, and flavors to make your diet interesting and nutritionally diverse.

Meal Planning:

Plan your meals ahead of time to ensure a balanced and diverse gut-friendly diet. This can help you incorporate a variety of ingredients and prevent monotony.

Listen to Your Body:

Pay attention to how your body responds to different foods. If certain ingredients or recipes don't agree with you, modify them or seek alternatives that work better for your digestive system.

Hydration is Key:

Don't forget the importance of staying hydrated. Water supports digestion and helps maintain a healthy gut environment.

Combine with a Healthy Lifestyle:

Remember that a gut health cookbook is just one aspect of supporting digestive wellness. Combine your gut-friendly meals with regular exercise, stress management, and sufficient sleep for overall well-being.

Always consult with a healthcare professional or nutritionist, especially if you have specific dietary concerns or health conditions. They can provide personalized advice based on your individual needs and circumstances.

Understanding gut health is essential for overall well-being, and a gut health cookbook serves as a valuable guide in fostering digestive wellness through nutrition.

The human gut is home to trillions of microorganisms collectively known as the gut microbiome, playing a crucial role in digestion, nutrient absorption, and immune function. A balanced and diverse microbiome is associated with numerous health benefits.

A gut health cookbook typically emphasizes ingredients that promote a thriving microbiome, such as probiotics, prebiotics, fiber-rich foods, and fermented delicacies.

These cookbooks provide insights into the intricate relationship between dietary choices and gut health, explaining how certain foods can either support or hinder the delicate balance of the microbiome.

These culinary guides often feature recipes that incorporate gut-friendly components, encouraging the consumption of whole foods, fruits, vegetables, and fermented delights. The recipes are designed not only for their nutritional value but also for their potential to enhance the diversity of the gut microbiome.

By following a gut health cookbook, individuals can adopt dietary practices that contribute to a healthier gut, potentially alleviating digestive issues and promoting overall vitality. However, it's important to approach these cookbooks with an understanding of one's unique dietary needs, consulting healthcare professionals for personalized advice on achieving and maintaining optimal gut health.

Principles Of Gut Health Cookbook

The principles of a gut health cookbook revolve around fostering a balanced and thriving gut microbiome, recognizing the pivotal role it plays in overall health.

These cookbooks are grounded in the idea that the gut is not merely a digestive organ but a complex ecosystem influenced by the foods we consume. The key principles include incorporating probiotics, prebiotics, and fiber-rich foods, all of which are instrumental in nurturing a diverse and resilient gut microbiome.

Probiotics, found in fermented foods like yogurt and kimchi, introduce beneficial bacteria to the gut, supporting digestion and immune function. Prebiotics, present in foods such as garlic and bananas, serve as nourishment for these beneficial bacteria. Meanwhile, fiber-rich foods like whole grains and vegetables promote digestive regularity and contribute to a flourishing gut environment.

Furthermore, a gut health cookbook often advocates for minimizing processed foods, sugars, and artificial additives that can disrupt the microbial balance.

Instead, the emphasis is on consuming nutrient-dense, whole foods to provide essential vitamins and minerals that contribute to overall gut well-being.

Benefits Of Gut Health Cookbook

A gut health cookbook offers a myriad of benefits that extend beyond the realm of culinary delights, focusing on promoting overall well-being through digestive wellness.

One of the primary advantages lies in the optimization of the gut microbiome. By incorporating recipes rich in probiotics and prebiotics, these cookbooks help maintain a diverse and balanced community of microorganisms in the gut.

This, in turn, supports efficient digestion, nutrient absorption, and bolsters the immune system.

These cookbooks often emphasize the consumption of whole, nutrient-dense foods, steering individuals away from processed and artificial ingredients.

The resulting dietary shift can lead to weight management, improved energy levels, and enhanced mental clarity.

Beyond physical health, gut health cookbooks may positively impact mental well-being. Emerging research suggests a strong connection between the gut and the brain, commonly referred to as the gut-brain axis.

A balanced gut microbiome is linked to improved mood, reduced stress levels, and better mental resilience.

Moreover, individuals grappling with digestive issues such as bloating or irregular bowel movements may find relief by following gut health cookbook principles.

These recipes often exclude common triggers for gastrointestinal discomfort, allowing individuals to identify and address potential food sensitivities.

In essence, a gut health cookbook serves as a holistic guide, fostering a harmonious relationship between the gut and the rest of the body, contributing to improved health, vitality, and a heightened sense of overall well-being

Tips For Gut Health Cookbook

Embarking on a journey to enhance gut health through a cookbook involves mindful choices and a commitment to nourishing the body from within. Here are some valuable tips for optimizing the benefits of a gut health cookbook:

Diverse Ingredients: Prioritize recipes that incorporate a variety of nutrient-dense and colorful fruits, vegetables, whole grains, and lean proteins. This diversity ensures a broad spectrum of essential nutrients for overall health.

Incorporate Fermented Foods: Embrace the power of fermentation by including foods like yogurt, kefir, sauerkraut, and kimchi. These probiotic-rich options introduce beneficial bacteria to the gut, supporting a flourishing microbiome.

Prioritize Prebiotics: Integrate prebiotic-rich foods such as garlic, onions, bananas, and asparagus. Prebiotics serve as food for the beneficial bacteria in the gut, fostering their growth and activity.

Mindful Cooking Techniques: Opt for cooking methods that preserve the nutritional integrity of ingredients. Steaming, sautéing, and baking are often preferable to frying, helping to retain essential vitamins and minerals.

Hydration: Stay well-hydrated, as water supports digestion and helps maintain a healthy gut environment. Herbal teas and infused water can be refreshing alternatives.

Moderation and Balance: Practice moderation with portion sizes and aim for a balanced distribution of macronutrients – carbohydrates, proteins, and healthy fats – in your meals.

Listen to Your Body: Pay attention to how your body responds to different foods. If certain ingredients cause discomfort, consider modifications or alternatives to cater to your individual digestive needs.

Meal Planning: Plan your meals in advance to ensure a consistent intake of gut-friendly foods. This can help you avoid reliance on processed or convenience foods.

By incorporating these tips into your culinary journey, a gut health cookbook becomes a powerful tool for promoting digestive wellness and overall health.

Guidelines For A Gut Health Cookbook

Navigating a gut health cookbook involves embracing guidelines that prioritize the well-being of your digestive system. Here are essential guidelines to maximize the benefits of such cookbooks:

Probiotic-Rich Choices: Select recipes featuring probiotic-rich foods like yogurt, kefir, kombucha, and fermented vegetables. Probiotics contribute to a balanced gut microbiome, supporting digestion and immune function.

Incorporate Fiber: Prioritize recipes abundant in fiber from whole grains, fruits, and vegetables. Fiber promotes regular bowel movements, aids in satiety, and fosters a diverse gut microbiome.

Prebiotic Power: Integrate prebiotic foods such as garlic, onions, leeks, and asparagus. These ingredients fuel the growth of beneficial gut bacteria, enhancing the overall health of the microbiome.

Mindful Cooking Techniques: Embrace cooking methods that preserve the nutritional integrity of ingredients. Steaming, baking, and sautéing retain essential nutrients, contributing to a wholesome and gut-friendly meal.

Hydration Habits: Prioritize hydration with water and herbal teas. Proper fluid intake supports digestion, ensuring a well-lubricated and healthy gut environment.

Limit Processed Foods: Minimize the consumption of processed and artificial additives. Opt for whole, natural foods to reduce the intake of potential gut irritants and enhance overall nutritional intake.

Balance Macronutrients: Strive for a balance of carbohydrates, proteins, and healthy fats in your meals. This helps maintain stable energy levels and supports overall nutritional needs.

Personalize for Sensitivities: Tailor recipes to accommodate individual sensitivities. Pay attention to how your body responds to certain ingredients, making modifications as needed to suit your digestive comfort.

By adhering to these guidelines, a gut health cookbook becomes a practical resource for cultivating a digestive environment that promotes overall well-being. These principles empower individuals to make informed dietary choices that positively impact their gut health and, consequently, their holistic health.

Causes Of Gut Health Disease

Gut health diseases can arise from a combination of genetic, environmental, and lifestyle factors. Understanding the various causes can provide insights into preventive measures and potential treatments:

Dietary Choices: Poor dietary habits, characterized by a high intake of processed foods, sugars, and low-fiber diets, can contribute to imbalances in the gut microbiome. Diets lacking in diverse, nutrient-rich foods may compromise the health of the digestive system.

Antibiotic Use: Prolonged or frequent use of antibiotics can disrupt the balance of the gut microbiota by indiscriminately killing both harmful and beneficial bacteria. This imbalance may lead to conditions like dysbiosis, affecting digestion and overall gut health.

Stress: Chronic stress can impact the gut-brain axis, influencing the function of the digestive system. Stress-related changes in gut motility, blood flow, and permeability may contribute to the development or exacerbation of gut health disorders.

Infections: Bacterial, viral, or parasitic infections can lead to inflammation and damage to the gastrointestinal tract, potentially causing conditions like gastroenteritis, inflammatory bowel disease (IBD), or irritable bowel syndrome (IBS).

Genetic Predisposition: Some individuals may have a genetic predisposition to certain gut health diseases, such as Crohn's disease or ulcerative colitis. Genetic factors can influence susceptibility to inflammation and immune responses within the digestive tract.

Lack of Physical Activity: Sedentary lifestyles may contribute to sluggish bowel movements and a compromised gut environment. Regular physical activity can support a healthy digestive system.

Environmental Factors: Exposure to environmental pollutants, toxins, and certain chemicals may adversely affect gut health. These factors can disrupt the balance of the gut microbiome and contribute to inflammation.

Age and Hormonal Changes: Aging and hormonal fluctuations, especially in women, can impact gut health. Menopausal changes, for example, may influence gut microbiota composition and contribute to gastrointestinal symptoms.

Understanding the multifaceted causes of gut health diseases underscores the importance of a holistic approach to digestive wellness, incorporating a balanced diet, stress management, regular physical activity, and appropriate medical interventions when necessary. Individuals experiencing persistent gut-related symptoms should consult with healthcare professionals for accurate diagnosis and tailored treatment plans.

Symptoms Of Gut Health Disease

Symptoms of gut health diseases can manifest in various ways, ranging from mild discomfort to severe disruptions in daily life. Recognizing these signs is crucial for early intervention and proper management. Common symptoms include:

Digestive Issues: Persistent and recurring digestive problems such as bloating, gas, abdominal pain, cramping, and irregular bowel movements may indicate underlying gut health issues. Conditions like irritable bowel syndrome (IBS) or inflammatory bowel disease (IBD) often present with these symptoms.

Changes in Bowel Habits: Persistent diarrhea, constipation, or alternating between the two can be indicative of gut health disorders. Unexplained changes in stool consistency or color may also raise concerns.

Fatigue: Chronic fatigue or a general feeling of lethargy can be associated with gut health problems. Malabsorption of nutrients due to digestive issues may contribute to low energy levels.

Food Intolerances: Developing sensitivities or intolerances to certain foods, accompanied by symptoms like nausea, vomiting, or diarrhea, may suggest compromised gut health.

Unexplained Weight Changes: Significant and unexplained weight loss or gain can be associated with various gut health conditions, including malabsorption issues, inflammatory disorders, or hormonal imbalances.

Skin Issues: Conditions like acne, eczema, or psoriasis may be linked to imbalances in the gut microbiome. The gut-skin connection underscores the importance of digestive health in maintaining overall well-being.

Joint Pain: Inflammatory conditions affecting the gut may also manifest as joint pain. Conditions like Crohn's disease or celiac disease may lead to inflammation that extends beyond the digestive tract.

Mood Disturbances: The gut-brain axis plays a crucial role in mental health. Gut health issues can contribute to mood disorders, including anxiety and depression. Brain fog and difficulty concentrating are also potential symptoms.

It's important to note that symptoms can vary widely, and individual experiences may differ. Persistent or severe symptoms should prompt consultation with healthcare professionals for a thorough evaluation, accurate diagnosis, and appropriate management of gut health conditions. Early detection and intervention can significantly improve outcomes and quality of life for individuals dealing with gut health issues.

Types Of Gut Health Disease

Gut health diseases encompass a spectrum of conditions affecting the gastrointestinal tract, each with unique characteristics and implications. Some notable types include:

Inflammatory Bowel Disease (IBD): Comprising Crohn's disease and ulcerative colitis, IBD involves chronic inflammation of the digestive tract. Symptoms include abdominal pain, diarrhea, weight loss, and fatigue.

Irritable Bowel Syndrome (IBS): IBS is a functional gastrointestinal disorder characterized by abdominal pain, bloating, and changes in bowel habits. It does not involve inflammation but can significantly impact quality of life.

Celiac Disease: An autoimmune condition triggered by gluten consumption, celiac disease causes damage to the small intestine. Symptoms include diarrhea, weight loss, and nutritional deficiencies.

Gastroesophageal Reflux Disease (GERD): GERD occurs when stomach acid frequently flows back into the esophagus, causing symptoms like heartburn, regurgitation, and chest pain.

Diverticulitis: This condition involves inflammation or infection of small pouches (diverticula) that can form in the walls of the colon. Symptoms may include abdominal pain, fever, and changes in bowel habits.

Gastroenteritis: Often caused by viral or bacterial infections, gastroenteritis leads to inflammation of the stomach and intestines. Symptoms include diarrhea, vomiting, and abdominal cramps.

Candida Overgrowth: An imbalance of the naturally occurring yeast Candida in the gut can lead to overgrowth. Symptoms may include digestive issues, fatigue, and skin problems.

Small Intestinal Bacterial Overgrowth (SIBO): SIBO involves an overgrowth of bacteria in the small intestine, leading to symptoms like bloating, gas, diarrhea, and malabsorption of nutrients.

Colorectal Cancer: Cancer affecting the colon or rectum, colorectal cancer can cause changes in bowel habits, blood in the stool, abdominal pain, and unintended weight loss.

Gallstones: While primarily affecting the gallbladder, gallstones can lead to digestive discomfort, especially after meals, and may require medical intervention.

These are just a few examples, and many other conditions can impact gut health. It's essential to consult healthcare professionals for accurate diagnosis and tailored treatment plans based on individual symptoms and medical history. Early detection and proper management are key in addressing gut health diseases effectively.

Risk Factors Of Gut Health Disease

Several risk factors contribute to the development of gut health diseases, highlighting the multifaceted nature of these conditions. Understanding these risk factors is crucial for prevention and early intervention. Common contributors include:

Genetic Predisposition: Family history plays a significant role in certain gut health diseases, such as inflammatory bowel disease (IBD) and celiac disease. Individuals with close relatives affected by these conditions may have an increased risk.

Dietary Choices: Diets high in processed foods, low in fiber, and lacking diversity can disrupt the balance of the gut microbiome, increasing the risk of conditions like irritable bowel syndrome (IBS) and colorectal cancer.

Antibiotic Use: Prolonged or frequent use of antibiotics can disturb the natural balance of bacteria in the gut, potentially leading to conditions like small intestinal bacterial overgrowth (SIBO) or Clostridium difficile infection.

Stress and Lifestyle Factors: Chronic stress, sedentary lifestyles, and inadequate sleep can negatively impact gut health. Stress, in particular, may contribute to conditions like gastroesophageal reflux disease (GERD) and irritable bowel syndrome (IBS).

Age: The risk of gut health diseases, such as colorectal cancer, increases with age. Regular screenings are recommended, especially for individuals over 50.

Autoimmune Conditions: Certain autoimmune disorders, such as rheumatoid arthritis or lupus, may increase the risk of developing gut-related conditions like inflammatory bowel disease.

Previous Gastrointestinal Surgery: Individuals with a history of gastrointestinal surgeries, such as bowel resection, may be at an increased risk of developing complications or altered gut function.

Environmental Exposures: Exposure to environmental pollutants, toxins, or infections may contribute to the development of gut health diseases. This can include factors such as contaminated water or exposure to specific pathogens.

Obesity: Being overweight or obese is associated with an increased risk of developing conditions like gallstones and non-alcoholic fatty liver disease, impacting overall gut health.

Smoking and Alcohol Consumption: Both smoking and excessive alcohol consumption have been linked to an elevated risk of various gut health issues, including esophageal and colorectal cancers.

GUT HEALTH RECIPES

BREAKFAST

1. Greek Yogurt Parfait:

Ingredients:

- ✓ 1 cup Greek yogurt (unsweetened)
- ✓ 1/2 cup mixed berries (blueberries, strawberries)
- ✓ 1 tablespoon chia seeds
- ✓ 1 tablespoon honey or maple syrup
- ✓ 1/4 cup granola (preferably low in added sugars)

Instructions:

- ✓ In a glass or bowl, layer Greek yogurt at the bottom.
- ✓ Add a layer of mixed berries.
- ✓ Sprinkle chia seeds over the berries.
- ✓ Drizzle honey or maple syrup on top.
- ✓ Finish with a layer of granola.
- ✓ Repeat for additional layers.
- ✓ Serve chilled.

Health Benefits:

- ✓ This parfait is rich in probiotics from Greek yogurt, high in fiber from chia seeds and granola, and provides antioxidants from berries. It supports gut health by promoting a diverse microbiome.

Preparation Time: 5 minutes

2. Avocado and Spinach Smoothie:

Ingredients:

- ✓ 1/2 avocado
- ✓ 1 cup spinach leaves
- ✓ 1/2 banana
- ✓ 1/2 cup almond milk (unsweetened)
- ✓ 1 tablespoon flaxseeds (ground)
- ✓ Ice cubes (optional)

Instructions:

- ✓ Blend avocado, spinach, banana, and almond milk until smooth.
- ✓ Add ground flaxseeds and blend again.
- ✓ Add ice cubes if desired and blend until well combined.
- ✓ Pour into a glass and enjoy immediately.

Health Benefits:

- ✓ This smoothie provides healthy fats from avocado, fiber from spinach and flaxseeds, and a good dose of vitamins and minerals. It supports gut health through its nutrient-rich ingredients.

Preparation Time: 5 minutes

3. Overnight Oats with Berries:

Ingredients:

- ✓ 1/2 cup rolled oats
- ✓ 1/2 cup Greek yogurt (unsweetened)
- ✓ 1/2 cup almond milk (unsweetened)
- ✓ 1/2 cup mixed berries
- ✓ 1 tablespoon chia seeds
- ✓ 1 teaspoon honey or maple syrup

Instructions:

- ✓ In a jar, combine rolled oats, Greek yogurt, almond milk, chia seeds, and honey.
- ✓ Stir well, ensuring oats are fully immersed in the liquid.
- ✓ Add mixed berries on top.
- ✓ Seal the jar and refrigerate overnight.
- ✓ In the morning, stir and enjoy.

Health Benefits:

- ✓ This breakfast is a great source of probiotics, fiber, and antioxidants, supporting gut health and providing sustained energy throughout the morning.

Preparation Time: 10 minutes (plus overnight soaking)

4. Quinoa Breakfast Bowl:

Ingredients:

- ✓ 1/2 cup cooked quinoa
- ✓ 1/4 cup sliced almonds
- ✓ 1/2 cup diced mango
- ✓ 1 tablespoon pumpkin seeds
- ✓ 1/2 cup coconut milk (unsweetened)
- ✓ 1 teaspoon honey or agave syrup

Instructions:

- ✓ In a bowl, combine cooked quinoa, sliced almonds, diced mango, and pumpkin seeds.
- ✓ Drizzle coconut milk over the mixture.
- ✓ Sweeten with honey or agave syrup.
- ✓ Mix well and enjoy.

Health Benefits:

- ✓ This bowl offers a blend of fiber, protein, and healthy fats, promoting gut health and providing a satisfying and nutrient-dense breakfast.

Preparation Time: 15 minutes (if quinoa is pre-cooked)

5. Berry and Spinach Breakfast Salad:

Ingredients:

- ✓ 2 cups fresh spinach leaves
- ✓ 1/2 cup mixed berries (blueberries, raspberries, strawberries)
- ✓ 1/4 cup walnuts, chopped
- ✓ 1/4 cup feta cheese, crumbled
- ✓ 1 tablespoon balsamic vinaigrette dressing

Instructions:

- ✓ In a bowl, combine fresh spinach, mixed berries, chopped walnuts, and crumbled feta cheese.
- ✓ Drizzle balsamic vinaigrette dressing over the salad.
- ✓ Toss gently to mix the ingredients.
- ✓ Serve immediately.

Health Benefits:

- ✓ This salad provides a mix of fiber, antioxidants, and omega-3 fatty acids from berries and walnuts. The spinach offers additional vitamins and minerals, supporting gut health and overall well-being.

Preparation Time: 7 minutes

6. Turmeric and Ginger Smoothie Bowl:

Ingredients:

- ✓ 1 frozen banana
- ✓ 1/2 cup pineapple chunks
- ✓ 1/2 teaspoon ground turmeric
- ✓ 1/2 teaspoon grated ginger
- ✓ 1 cup coconut water
- ✓ Toppings: sliced kiwi, shredded coconut, chia seeds

Instructions:

- ✓ Blend frozen banana, pineapple chunks, turmeric, ginger, and coconut water until smooth.
- ✓ Pour the smoothie into a bowl.
- ✓ Top with sliced kiwi, shredded coconut, and chia seeds.
- ✓ Enjoy with a spoon.

Health Benefits:

- ✓ This smoothie bowl incorporates anti-inflammatory ingredients like turmeric and ginger, along with hydrating coconut water. It supports gut health and provides a refreshing start to the day.

Preparation Time: 8 minutes

7. Whole Grain Toast with Smashed Avocado and Radishes:

Ingredients:

- ✓ 2 slices whole-grain bread
- ✓ 1 ripe avocado, smashed
- ✓ 4 radishes, thinly sliced
- ✓ 1 tablespoon olive oil
- ✓ Sprinkle of sea salt and black pepper
- ✓ Fresh lemon juice (optional)

Instructions:

- ✓ Toast whole-grain bread slices to your liking.
- ✓ Spread smashed avocado evenly over each slice.
- ✓ Arrange thinly sliced radishes on top.
- ✓ Drizzle olive oil over the toast and sprinkle with sea salt and black pepper.
- ✓ Optionally, squeeze fresh lemon juice for added zest.
- ✓ Serve immediately.

Health Benefits:

- ✓ This breakfast option offers a combination of whole grains, healthy fats from avocado, and the crisp freshness of radishes. It's rich in fiber and provides a satisfying and nutritious morning meal.

Preparation Time: 10 minutes

8. Chia Seed Pudding with Mixed Berries:

Ingredients:

- ✓ 3 tablespoons chia seeds
- ✓ 1 cup almond milk (unsweetened)
- ✓ 1/2 teaspoon vanilla extract
- ✓ 1 tablespoon maple syrup or honey
- ✓ 1/2 cup mixed berries (strawberries, blueberries, raspberries)

Instructions:

- ✓ In a bowl, mix chia seeds, almond milk, vanilla extract, and maple syrup.
- ✓ Stir well and let it sit for 5 minutes.
- ✓ Stir again to prevent clumping and refrigerate for at least 2 hours or overnight.
- ✓ Before serving, layer the chia pudding with mixed berries.
- ✓ Garnish with additional berries on top.
- ✓ Enjoy this nutritious and gut-friendly pudding.

Health Benefits:

- ✓ Chia seeds provide omega-3 fatty acids and fiber, while berries offer antioxidants. This pudding is gentle on the stomach and supports digestive health.

Preparation Time: 5 minutes (plus chilling time)

9. Sweet Potato and Kale Breakfast Hash:

Ingredients:

- ✓ 1 medium sweet potato, diced
- ✓ 1 cup kale, chopped
- ✓ 1/2 onion, finely chopped
- ✓ 1 clove garlic, minced
- ✓ 2 eggs
- ✓ 1 tablespoon olive oil
- ✓ Salt and pepper to taste

Instructions:

- ✓ Heat olive oil in a skillet over medium heat.
- ✓ Add diced sweet potato and cook until slightly browned and softened.
- ✓ Add chopped onion and garlic, sauté until fragrant.
- ✓ Stir in kale and cook until wilted.
- ✓ Create wells in the mixture and crack eggs into them.
- ✓ Cover and cook until eggs are done to your liking.
- ✓ Season with salt and pepper, then serve.

Health Benefits:

✓ This breakfast hash is rich in fiber from sweet potatoes and kale, providing a hearty and nutritious option that supports gut health and offers a balance of vitamins and minerals.

Preparation Time: 20 minutes

10. Oat Bran Porridge with Apples and Cinnamon:

Ingredients:

✓ 1/2 cup oat bran
✓ 1 1/2 cups water or milk of choice
✓ 1 apple, diced
✓ 1/2 teaspoon cinnamon
✓ 1 tablespoon honey or maple syrup
✓ Nuts or seeds for topping (optional)

Instructions:

✓ In a saucepan, bring water or milk to a boil.
✓ Stir in oat bran and reduce heat to low. Cook until thickened.
✓ Add diced apples, cinnamon, and sweeten with honey or maple syrup.
✓ Continue cooking until apples are tender and flavors meld.
✓ Top with nuts or seeds if desired.
✓ Serve warm.

Health Benefits:

- ✓ Oat bran is rich in soluble fiber, promoting digestive health. Apples provide additional fiber and antioxidants, while cinnamon adds flavor without added sugars.

Preparation Time: 15 minutes

LUNCH GUT HEALTH RECIPES

1. Quinoa and Vegetable Buddha Bowl:

Ingredients:

- ✓ 1 cup cooked quinoa
- ✓ 1 cup mixed vegetables (broccoli, bell peppers, carrots)
- ✓ 1/2 cup chickpeas (canned or cooked)
- ✓ 1 tablespoon olive oil
- ✓ 1 teaspoon lemon juice
- ✓ Salt and pepper to taste
- ✓ Optional toppings: avocado, pumpkin seeds

Instructions:

- ✓ In a pan, sauté mixed vegetables in olive oil until tender.
- ✓ Add cooked quinoa and chickpeas to the pan, stirring well.
- ✓ Drizzle with lemon juice and season with salt and pepper.
- ✓ Divide into bowls and top with avocado slices and pumpkin seeds if desired.
- ✓ Serve warm

Health Benefits:

✓ This bowl provides a blend of fiber, plant-based protein, and healthy fats, supporting gut health and offering a nutrient-dense and satisfying lunch.

Preparation Time: 20 minutes

2. Lentil and Kale Soup:

Ingredients:

✓ 1 cup dried lentils, rinsed

✓ 1 onion, diced

✓ 2 carrots, sliced

✓ 2 celery stalks, chopped

✓ 3 cups kale, chopped

✓ 4 cups vegetable broth

✓ 2 cloves garlic, minced

✓ 1 teaspoon cumin

✓ Salt and pepper to taste

✓ Olive oil for sautéing

Instructions:

✓ In a large pot, sauté onion, carrots, and celery in olive oil until softened.

✓ Add minced garlic and cumin, cooking for an additional minute.

✓ Pour in vegetable broth and add lentils. Bring to a boil, then reduce heat and simmer until lentils are tender.

✓ Stir in chopped kale and cook until wilted.

✓ Season with salt and pepper to taste.

✓ Ladle into bowls and serve.

Health Benefits:

✓ This soup is rich in fiber from lentils and kale, providing essential nutrients, antioxidants, and supporting digestive health.

Preparation Time: 30 minutes

3. Grilled Salmon with Quinoa and Asparagus:

Ingredients:

✓ 2 salmon fillets

✓ 1 cup quinoa, cooked

✓ 1 bunch asparagus, trimmed

✓ 1 lemon, sliced

✓ 2 tablespoons olive oil

✓ Fresh dill for garnish

✓ Salt and pepper to taste

Instructions:

✓ Preheat the grill. Season salmon fillets with salt, pepper, and a drizzle of olive oil.

✓ Grill salmon for 4-5 minutes per side or until cooked through.

✓ Toss asparagus with olive oil, salt, and pepper. Grill until tender.

✓ Arrange cooked quinoa, grilled salmon, and asparagus on plates.

✓ Garnish with lemon slices and fresh dill.

✓ Serve immediately.

Health Benefits:

✓ This dish provides omega-3 fatty acids from salmon, fiber from quinoa, and a variety of nutrients from asparagus, promoting gut health and overall well-being.

Preparation Time: 25 minutes

4. Chickpea and Vegetable Stir-Fry:

Ingredients:

✓ 1 can chickpeas, drained and rinsed

✓ 2 cups mixed vegetables (bell peppers, broccoli, snap peas)

✓ 1 cup quinoa, cooked

✓ 3 tablespoons soy sauce (low-sodium)

✓ 1 tablespoon sesame oil

✓ 2 cloves garlic, minced

✓ 1 teaspoon ginger, grated

✓ Green onions for garnish

✓ Sesame seeds for topping

Instructions:

✓ In a wok or skillet, heat sesame oil and sauté garlic and ginger until fragrant.

✓ Add mixed vegetables and stir-fry until slightly tender.

✓ Add chickpeas and cook until heated through.

✓ Stir in cooked quinoa and soy sauce, mixing well.

✓ Garnish with green onions and sesame seeds.

✓ Serve hot.

Health Benefits:

✓ This stir-fry is rich in plant-based protein from chickpeas, fiber from vegetables, and provides a variety of nutrients supporting gut health and digestive function.

Preparation Time: 20 minutes

5. Miso Glazed Tofu Bowl:

Ingredients:

✓ 1 cup firm tofu, cubed

✓ 2 tablespoons miso paste

✓ 1 tablespoon soy sauce (low-sodium)

✓ 1 tablespoon rice vinegar

✓ 1 tablespoon sesame oil

- ✓ 1 cup quinoa, cooked

- ✓ 1 cup steamed broccoli

- ✓ 1 carrot, julienned

- ✓ Sesame seeds for garnish

- ✓ Green onions for garnish

Instructions:

- ✓ In a bowl, mix miso paste, soy sauce, rice vinegar, and sesame oil to create the glaze.

- ✓ Toss cubed tofu in the glaze until well-coated.

- ✓ Bake tofu in the oven at 400°F (200°C) for 20-25 minutes or until golden.

- ✓ Assemble bowls with cooked quinoa, steamed broccoli, julienned carrots, and baked miso-glazed tofu.

- ✓ Garnish with sesame seeds and green onions.

- ✓ Serve warm.

Health Benefits:

- ✓ This tofu bowl provides plant-based protein, probiotics from miso, and a mix of fiber and vitamins from quinoa and vegetables, supporting gut health.

Preparation Time: 30 minutes

6. Rainbow Salad with Turmeric Dressing:

Ingredients:

- ✓ 2 cups mixed greens (spinach, kale, arugula)
- ✓ 1/2 cup shredded red cabbage
- ✓ 1/2 cup shredded carrots
- ✓ 1 bell pepper, thinly sliced
- ✓ 1 cucumber, diced
- ✓ 1/4 cup pumpkin seeds
- ✓ Dressing: 2 tablespoons olive oil, 1 tablespoon apple cider vinegar, 1 teaspoon turmeric, salt, and pepper to taste

Instructions:

- ✓ In a large bowl, combine mixed greens, shredded red cabbage, shredded carrots, sliced bell pepper, and diced cucumber.
- ✓ In a small bowl, whisk together olive oil, apple cider vinegar, turmeric, salt, and pepper to create the dressing.
- ✓ Drizzle the dressing over the salad and toss until well-coated.
- ✓ Sprinkle pumpkin seeds on top.
- ✓ Serve immediately.

Health Benefits:

- ✓ This vibrant salad offers a spectrum of nutrients, antioxidants, and anti-inflammatory properties from turmeric, supporting overall health and gut function.

Preparation Time: 15 minutes

7. Cauliflower Rice Stir-Fry with Shrimp:

Ingredients:

- ✓ 1-pound shrimp, peeled and deveined
- ✓ 3 cups cauliflower rice
- ✓ 1 cup snap peas, trimmed
- ✓ 1 red bell pepper, sliced
- ✓ 2 tablespoons coconut aminos (or soy sauce)
- ✓ 1 tablespoon olive oil
- ✓ 2 cloves garlic, minced
- ✓ 1 teaspoon ginger, grated
- ✓ Fresh cilantro for garnish
- ✓ Lime wedges for serving

Instructions:

- ✓ In a large pan, heat olive oil and sauté garlic and ginger until fragrant.
- ✓ Add shrimp and cook until pink and opaque.

- ✓ Add snap peas and bell pepper, stir-frying until vegetables are tender-crisp.
- ✓ Stir in cauliflower rice and coconut aminos, mixing well.
- ✓ Cook for an additional 3-4 minutes until everything is heated through.
- ✓ Garnish with fresh cilantro and serve with lime wedges.

Health Benefits:

- ✓ This stir-fry offers a low-carb option with cauliflower rice, lean protein from shrimp, and a variety of vegetables, promoting gut health and providing a delicious lunch option.

Preparation Time: 25 minutes

8. Chickpea and Spinach Stuffed Sweet Potatoes:

Ingredients:

- ✓ 2 medium sweet potatoes
- ✓ 1 can chickpeas, drained and rinsed
- ✓ 2 cups fresh spinach, chopped
- ✓ 1 red onion, finely chopped
- ✓ 2 cloves garlic, minced
- ✓ 1 teaspoon cumin
- ✓ 1 teaspoon paprika
- ✓ 1 tablespoon olive oil
- ✓ Salt and pepper to taste

✓ Greek yogurt for topping (optional)

Instructions:

✓ Preheat the oven to 400°F (200°C).

✓ Scrub sweet potatoes, pierce with a fork, and bake for 45-60 minutes until tender.

✓ In a pan, sauté chopped onion and garlic in olive oil until softened.

✓ Add chickpeas, spinach, cumin, paprika, salt, and pepper. Cook until spinach wilts.

✓ Cut open the sweet potatoes, fluff the flesh with a fork, and top with the chickpea-spinach mixture.

✓ Optionally, add a dollop of Greek yogurt on top.

✓ Serve warm.

Health Benefits:

✓ This dish combines the fiber from sweet potatoes and chickpeas with the iron and vitamins from spinach, offering a nutritious and gut-friendly lunch.

Preparation Time: 75 minutes

9. Mediterranean Quinoa Salad:

Ingredients:

✓ 1 cup quinoa, cooked

✓ 1 cup cherry tomatoes, halved

- ✓ 1 cucumber, diced
- ✓ 1/2 red onion, finely chopped
- ✓ 1/2 cup Kalamata olives, sliced
- ✓ 1/2 cup feta cheese, crumbled
- ✓ 3 tablespoons extra-virgin olive oil
- ✓ 2 tablespoons red wine vinegar
- ✓ 1 teaspoon dried oregano
- ✓ Salt and pepper to taste
- ✓ Fresh parsley for garnish

Instructions:

- ✓ In a large bowl, combine cooked quinoa, cherry tomatoes, cucumber, red onion, olives, and feta cheese.
- ✓ In a small bowl, whisk together olive oil, red wine vinegar, dried oregano, salt, and pepper to create the dressing.
- ✓ Pour the dressing over the salad and toss until well-coated.
- ✓ Garnish with fresh parsley.
- ✓ Serve chilled or at room temperature.

Health Benefits:

- ✓ This Mediterranean-inspired salad provides a mix of fiber, healthy fats, and antioxidants, supporting gut health and offering a flavorful and refreshing lunch option.

Preparation Time: 20 minutes

10. Broccoli and Salmon Quiche:

Ingredients:

- ✓ 1 pre-made whole wheat pie crust
- ✓ 1 cup broccoli florets, steamed
- ✓ 1/2 pound cooked salmon, flaked
- ✓ 1 cup cherry tomatoes, halved
- ✓ 4 large eggs
- ✓ 1 cup milk (dairy or plant-based)
- ✓ 1/2 cup feta cheese, crumbled
- ✓ Salt and pepper to taste
- ✓ Fresh dill for garnish

Instructions:

- ✓ Preheat the oven to 375°F (190°C).
- ✓ In the pie crust, evenly distribute steamed broccoli, flaked salmon, and cherry tomatoes.
- ✓ In a bowl, whisk together eggs, milk, feta cheese, salt, and pepper.
- ✓ Pour the egg mixture over the ingredients in the pie crust.
- ✓ Bake for 35-40 minutes or until the quiche is set and golden brown.
- ✓ Garnish with fresh dill.
- ✓ Allow to cool slightly before slicing and serving.

Health Benefits:

- ✓ This quiche provides omega-3 fatty acids from salmon, fiber from broccoli, and a variety of nutrients, making it a wholesome and gut-friendly lunch option.

Preparation Time: 50 minutes

DINNER GUT HEALTH RECIPE

1. Garlic Ginger Salmon with Roasted Vegetables:

Ingredients:

- ✓ 2 salmon fillets
- ✓ 2 tablespoons olive oil
- ✓ 2 cloves garlic, minced
- ✓ 1 tablespoon grated ginger
- ✓ 1 teaspoon soy sauce (low-sodium)
- ✓ 1 tablespoon honey
- ✓ Salt and pepper to taste
- ✓ 2 cups mixed vegetables (broccoli, bell peppers, carrots)
- ✓ Cooking spray or additional olive oil

Instructions:

- ✓ Preheat the oven to 400°F (200°C).
- ✓ In a small bowl, mix olive oil, minced garlic, grated ginger, soy sauce, honey, salt, and pepper to make the marinade.

✓ Place salmon fillets in a shallow dish and coat with the marinade. Let it marinate for 15-30 minutes.

✓ Meanwhile, toss mixed vegetables with a drizzle of olive oil, salt, and pepper on a baking sheet.

✓ Arrange marinated salmon fillets and vegetables on the baking sheet.

✓ Roast in the preheated oven for 15-20 minutes, or until the salmon is cooked through and vegetables are tender.

✓ Serve hot.

Health Benefits:

✓ This dish is rich in omega-3 fatty acids from salmon, antioxidants from garlic and ginger, and fiber from vegetables, promoting gut health and overall well-being.

Preparation Time: 30 minutes

2. Quinoa Stuffed Bell Peppers:

Ingredients:

✓ 4 large bell peppers

✓ 1 cup quinoa, cooked

✓ 1 can black beans, drained and rinsed

✓ 1 cup corn kernels (fresh or frozen)

✓ 1 cup diced tomatoes

✓ 1/2 cup diced red onion

- ✓ 2 cloves garlic, minced
- ✓ 1 teaspoon cumin
- ✓ 1 teaspoon paprika
- ✓ Salt and pepper to taste
- ✓ Fresh cilantro for garnish

Instructions:

- ✓ Preheat the oven to 375°F (190°C).
- ✓ Cut the tops off the bell peppers and remove seeds and membranes.
- ✓ In a large bowl, mix cooked quinoa, black beans, corn, diced tomatoes, red onion, minced garlic, cumin, paprika, salt, and pepper.
- ✓ Stuff the bell peppers with the quinoa mixture and place them in a baking dish.
- ✓ Cover the dish with foil and bake for 25-30 minutes, or until the peppers are tender.
- ✓ Garnish with fresh cilantro before serving.

Health Benefits:

- ✓ These stuffed bell peppers are packed with fiber, protein, and various vitamins and minerals, supporting gut health and providing a satisfying and nutritious dinner option.

Preparation Time: 45 minutes

3. Lemon Herb Chicken with Roasted Brussels Sprouts:

Ingredients:

- ✓ 2 boneless, skinless chicken breasts
- ✓ 2 tablespoons olive oil
- ✓ 2 tablespoons fresh lemon juice
- ✓ 2 cloves garlic, minced
- ✓ 1 teaspoon dried thyme
- ✓ 1 teaspoon dried rosemary
- ✓ Salt and pepper to taste
- ✓ 2 cups Brussels sprouts, trimmed and halved
- ✓ Cooking spray or additional olive oil

Instructions:

- ✓ Preheat the oven to 400°F (200°C).
- ✓ In a small bowl, whisk together olive oil, lemon juice, minced garlic, dried thyme, dried rosemary, salt, and pepper to create the marinade.
- ✓ Place chicken breasts in a shallow dish and coat with the marinade. Let it marinate for 15-30 minutes.
- ✓ Meanwhile, toss Brussels sprouts with a drizzle of olive oil, salt, and pepper on a baking sheet.

- ✓ Arrange marinated chicken breasts and Brussels sprouts on the baking sheet.
- ✓ Roast in the preheated oven for 25-30 minutes, or until the chicken is cooked through and Brussels sprouts are tender and caramelized.
- ✓ Serve hot.

Health Benefits:

- ✓ This dish provides lean protein from chicken, fiber from Brussels sprouts, and a boost of flavor from herbs and lemon, supporting gut health and offering a delicious dinner option.

Preparation Time: 40 minutes

4. Lentil and Vegetable Curry:

Ingredients:

- ✓ 1 cup dried lentils, rinsed
- ✓ 2 cups vegetable broth
- ✓ 1 tablespoon olive oil
- ✓ 1 onion, diced
- ✓ 2 cloves garlic, minced
- ✓ 1 tablespoon grated ginger
- ✓ 2 carrots, diced
- ✓ 2 potatoes, diced
- ✓ 1 can coconut milk

- ✓ 2 tablespoons curry powder
- ✓ Salt and pepper to taste
- ✓ Fresh cilantro for garnish

Instructions:

- ✓ In a large pot, heat olive oil over medium heat. Add diced onion, minced garlic, and grated ginger, cooking until softened and fragrant.
- ✓ Add diced carrots and potatoes to the pot, stirring well.
- ✓ Pour in vegetable broth and add rinsed lentils. Bring to a boil, then reduce heat and simmer until lentils and vegetables are tender.
- ✓ Stir in coconut milk and curry powder, mixing well. Simmer for an additional 5-10 minutes to allow flavors to meld.
- ✓ Season with salt and pepper to taste.
- ✓ Garnish with fresh cilantro before serving.
- ✓ Serve hot with rice or naan bread.

Health Benefits:

- ✓ This lentil and vegetable curry is rich in fiber, plant-based protein, and various vitamins and minerals, supporting gut health and providing a hearty and flavorful dinner option.

Preparation Time: 45 minutes

5. Baked Sweet Potato and Black Bean Casserole:

Ingredients:

- ✓ 2 large sweet potatoes, peeled and sliced
- ✓ 1 can black beans, drained and rinsed
- ✓ 1 cup corn kernels (fresh or frozen)
- ✓ 1 red bell pepper, diced
- ✓ 1 cup diced tomatoes
- ✓ 1 cup shredded cheddar cheese
- ✓ 1 teaspoon cumin
- ✓ 1 teaspoon chili powder
- ✓ Salt and pepper to taste
- ✓ Olive oil for drizzling
- ✓ Fresh cilantro for garnish

Instructions:

- ✓ Preheat the oven to 375°F (190°C).
- ✓ In a baking dish, layer sliced sweet potatoes, black beans, corn, red bell pepper, and diced tomatoes.
- ✓ Sprinkle cumin, chili powder, salt, and pepper over the layers.
- ✓ Drizzle olive oil over the top and cover the dish with foil.
- ✓ Bake for 30-35 minutes or until sweet potatoes are tender.

✓ Remove the foil, sprinkle shredded cheddar cheese over the casserole, and bake for an additional 10 minutes until the cheese is melted and bubbly.

✓ Garnish with fresh cilantro before serving.

Health Benefits:

✓ This casserole is rich in fiber, antioxidants, and vitamins from sweet potatoes and vegetables, supporting gut health and offering a satisfying and comforting dinner option.

Preparation Time: 50 minutes

6. Quinoa and Kale Stuffed Acorn Squash:

Ingredients:

✓ 2 acorn squash, halved and seeds removed

✓ 1 cup quinoa, cooked

✓ 2 cups kale, chopped

✓ 1/2 cup dried cranberries

✓ 1/4 cup pecans, chopped

✓ 1 tablespoon olive oil

✓ 1 tablespoon balsamic vinegar

✓ Salt and pepper to taste

✓ Goat cheese for topping (optional)

Instructions:

✓ Preheat the oven to 400°F (200°C).

- ✓ Place acorn squash halves on a baking sheet, cut side up.

- ✓ In a bowl, mix cooked quinoa, chopped kale, dried cranberries, chopped pecans, olive oil, balsamic vinegar, salt, and pepper.

- ✓ Stuff each acorn squash half with the quinoa mixture.

- ✓ Bake for 30-35 minutes or until the squash is tender.

- ✓ Optionally, crumble goat cheese on top before serving.

Health Benefits:

- ✓ This dish provides a combination of fiber, vitamins, and minerals from quinoa, kale, and acorn squash, supporting gut health and offering a nutrient-dense dinner option.

Preparation Time: 45 minutes

7. Turmeric Chicken and Vegetable Stir-Fry:

Ingredients:

- ✓ 2 boneless, skinless chicken breasts, thinly sliced

- ✓ 2 tablespoons olive oil

- ✓ 1 tablespoon turmeric powder

- ✓ 1 tablespoon soy sauce (low-sodium)

- ✓ 1 tablespoon honey

- ✓ 1 bell pepper, thinly sliced

- ✓ 1 zucchini, sliced

- ✓ 1 cup broccoli florets

- ✓ 2 cloves garlic, minced
- ✓ 1 tablespoon grated ginger
- ✓ Sesame seeds for garnish
- ✓ Green onions for garnish
- ✓ Brown rice for serving

Instructions:

- ✓ In a bowl, mix sliced chicken with turmeric, soy sauce, and honey. Let it marinate for 15-30 minutes.
- ✓ Heat olive oil in a wok or skillet over medium-high heat.
- ✓ Add marinated chicken and cook until browned and cooked through.
- ✓ Add sliced bell pepper, zucchini, broccoli, minced garlic, and grated ginger. Stir-fry until vegetables are tender-crisp.
- ✓ Garnish with sesame seeds and green onions.
- ✓ Serve over cooked brown rice.

Health Benefits:

- ✓ This stir-fry is rich in anti-inflammatory properties from turmeric, lean protein from chicken, and a variety of vegetables, supporting gut health and providing a quick and flavorful dinner option.

Preparation Time: 30 minutes

8. Spaghetti Squash with Turkey Bolognese:

Ingredients:

- ✓ 1 large spaghetti squash, halved and seeds removed
- ✓ 1 pound ground turkey
- ✓ 1 can crushed tomatoes
- ✓ 1 onion, diced
- ✓ 2 cloves garlic, minced
- ✓ 1 teaspoon dried oregano
- ✓ 1 teaspoon dried basil
- ✓ Salt and pepper to taste
- ✓ Olive oil for sautéing
- ✓ Fresh parsley for garnish
- ✓ Grated Parmesan cheese for topping

Instructions:

- ✓ Preheat the oven to 400°F (200°C).
- ✓ Place spaghetti squash halves on a baking sheet, cut side up.
- ✓ Drizzle with olive oil, salt, and pepper. Roast for 40-45 minutes or until squash is tender.
- ✓ In a skillet, sauté diced onion and minced garlic in olive oil until softened.
- ✓ Add ground turkey and cook until browned.
- ✓ Stir in crushed tomatoes, dried oregano, dried basil, salt, and pepper. Simmer for 15-20 minutes.

- ✓ Scrape the spaghetti squash with a fork to create "noodles" and serve topped with turkey Bolognese.
- ✓ Garnish with fresh parsley and grated Parmesan.

Health Benefits:

- ✓ This dish offers a low-carb alternative using spaghetti squash, lean protein from turkey, and a rich source of vitamins and minerals, supporting gut health and providing a wholesome dinner.

Preparation Time: 70 minutes

9. Ginger-Lime Tofu Stir-Fry:

Ingredients:

- ✓ 1 block firm tofu, pressed and cubed
- ✓ 2 tablespoons soy sauce (low-sodium)
- ✓ 1 tablespoon sesame oil
- ✓ 1 tablespoon rice vinegar
- ✓ 1 tablespoon fresh ginger, grated
- ✓ Zest and juice of 1 lime
- ✓ 2 tablespoons olive oil
- ✓ 1 bell pepper, sliced
- ✓ 1 cup snap peas, trimmed
- ✓ 2 carrots, julienned
- ✓ Brown rice for serving

Instructions:

- ✓ In a bowl, mix cubed tofu with soy sauce, sesame oil, rice vinegar, grated ginger, lime zest, and lime juice. Let it marinate for 15-30 minutes.
- ✓ Heat olive oil in a wok or skillet over medium-high heat.
- ✓ Add marinated tofu and cook until browned on all sides.
- ✓ Add sliced bell pepper, snap peas, and julienned carrots. Stir-fry until vegetables are tender-crisp.
- ✓ Serve the ginger-lime tofu stir-fry over cooked brown rice.

Health Benefits:

- ✓ This stir-fry offers plant-based protein from tofu, anti-inflammatory benefits from ginger and lime, and a variety of vegetables, promoting gut health and providing a light and flavorful dinner option.

Preparation Time: 40 minutes

10. Mediterranean Chickpea Salad:

Ingredients:

- ✓ 2 cans chickpeas, drained and rinsed
- ✓ 1 cucumber, diced
- ✓ 1 cup cherry tomatoes, halved
- ✓ 1/2 red onion, finely chopped
- ✓ 1/2 cup Kalamata olives, sliced

- ✓ 1/2 cup feta cheese, crumbled
- ✓ 3 tablespoons extra-virgin olive oil
- ✓ 2 tablespoons red wine vinegar
- ✓ 1 teaspoon dried oregano
- ✓ Salt and pepper to taste
- ✓ Fresh parsley for garnish

Instructions:

- ✓ In a large bowl, combine chickpeas, diced cucumber, cherry tomatoes, chopped red onion, sliced Kalamata olives, and crumbled feta cheese.
- ✓ In a small bowl, whisk together olive oil, red wine vinegar, dried oregano, salt, and pepper to create the dressing.
- ✓ Pour the dressing over the salad and toss until well-coated.
- ✓ Garnish with fresh parsley.
- ✓ Serve chilled.

Health Benefits:

- ✓ This Mediterranean-inspired salad provides a mix of fiber, healthy fats, and antioxidants, supporting gut health and offering a refreshing and nutritious dinner option.

Preparation Time: 15 minutes

1. Berry and Almond Butter Smoothie Bowl:

Ingredients:

- ✓ 1 cup mixed berries (strawberries, blueberries, raspberries)
- ✓ 1 banana, frozen
- ✓ 1/2 cup almond milk (unsweetened)
- ✓ 1 tablespoon almond butter
- ✓ Toppings: granola, chia seeds, sliced almonds

Instructions:

- ✓ In a blender, combine mixed berries, frozen banana, almond milk, and almond butter.
- ✓ Blend until smooth and creamy.
- ✓ Pour the smoothie into a bowl.
- ✓ Top with granola, chia seeds, and sliced almonds.
- ✓ Enjoy with a spoon.

Health Benefits:

- ✓ This smoothie bowl is rich in antioxidants from berries, provides healthy fats and protein from almond butter, and offers fiber from the added toppings, supporting gut health and providing sustained energy.

Preparation Time: 10 minutes

2. Greek Yogurt and Cucumber Dip with Whole Grain Crackers:

Ingredients:

- ✓ 1 cup Greek yogurt (unsweetened)
- ✓ 1/2 cucumber, finely diced
- ✓ 1 clove garlic, minced
- ✓ 1 tablespoon fresh dill, chopped
- ✓ 1 tablespoon lemon juice
- ✓ Whole grain crackers for serving

Instructions:

- ✓ In a bowl, combine Greek yogurt, diced cucumber, minced garlic, chopped dill, and lemon juice.
- ✓ Mix well until ingredients are evenly distributed.
- ✓ Refrigerate for at least 30 minutes to allow flavors to meld.
- ✓ Serve with whole grain crackers.

Health Benefits:

- ✓ This snack provides probiotics from Greek yogurt, hydration and fiber from cucumber, and anti-inflammatory properties from fresh dill, contributing to a healthy gut.

Preparation Time: 15 minutes

3. Roasted Chickpeas with Turmeric and Cumin:

Ingredients:

- ✓ 1 can chickpeas, drained and rinsed
- ✓ 1 tablespoon olive oil
- ✓ 1 teaspoon turmeric
- ✓ 1 teaspoon cumin
- ✓ 1/2 teaspoon smoked paprika
- ✓ Salt and pepper to taste

Instructions:

- ✓ Preheat the oven to 400°F (200°C).
- ✓ Pat the chickpeas dry with a paper towel.
- ✓ In a bowl, toss chickpeas with olive oil, turmeric, cumin, smoked paprika, salt, and pepper.
- ✓ Spread the chickpeas on a baking sheet in a single layer.
- ✓ Roast in the oven for 25-30 minutes or until golden and crispy.
- ✓ Allow to cool before serving.

Health Benefits:

- ✓ Roasted chickpeas offer a crunchy and fiber-rich snack. Turmeric and cumin provide anti-inflammatory benefits, contributing to gut health.

Preparation Time: 35 minutes

4. Apple and Almond Butter Rice Cakes:

Ingredients:

- ✓ 2 rice cakes (whole grain or brown rice)
- ✓ 2 tablespoons almond butter
- ✓ 1 apple, thinly sliced
- ✓ 1 tablespoon pumpkin seeds
- ✓ Drizzle of honey (optional)

Instructions:

- ✓ Spread almond butter evenly over each rice cake.
- ✓ Top with thinly sliced apple.
- ✓ Sprinkle pumpkin seeds on top.
- ✓ Optionally, drizzle honey for added sweetness.
- ✓ Serve immediately.

Health Benefits:

- ✓ This snack combines the fiber from rice cakes and apple, the protein and healthy fats from almond butter, and the nutritional benefits of pumpkin seeds, promoting gut health and providing a satisfying treat.

Preparation Time: 5 minutes

5. Hummus and Veggie Stuffed Bell Peppers:

Ingredients:

- ✓ 1 cup hummus (homemade or store-bought)
- ✓ 2 bell peppers (red, yellow, or green)
- ✓ Assorted veggies for stuffing (carrots, cucumber, cherry tomatoes)
- ✓ Fresh herbs for garnish (parsley, cilantro)
- ✓ Whole grain pita bread or cucumber slices for serving

Instructions:

- ✓ Wash and cut bell peppers into strips.
- ✓ Fill each strip with hummus.
- ✓ Slice assorted veggies into matchsticks and stuff them into the hummus-filled bell pepper strips.
- ✓ Garnish with fresh herbs.
- ✓ Serve with whole grain pita bread or cucumber slices.

Health Benefits:

- ✓ This snack is rich in fiber from veggies, provides plant-based protein from hummus, and offers a variety of vitamins and minerals, supporting gut health and providing a satisfying crunch.

Preparation Time: 10 minutes

6. Chia Seed Pudding with Mango Puree:

Ingredients:

- ✓ 3 tablespoons chia seeds
- ✓ 1 cup almond milk (unsweetened)
- ✓ 1 ripe mango, peeled and diced
- ✓ 1 teaspoon honey or maple syrup
- ✓ Fresh mint leaves for garnish

Instructions:

- ✓ In a bowl, mix chia seeds and almond milk. Let it sit for 5 minutes.
- ✓ Stir again to prevent clumping and refrigerate for at least 2 hours or overnight.
- ✓ In a blender, puree diced mango until smooth.
- ✓ Layer chia pudding with mango puree in serving glasses.
- ✓ Drizzle honey or maple syrup on top.
- ✓ Garnish with fresh mint leaves.

Health Benefits:

- ✓ Chia seeds provide omega-3 fatty acids and fiber, while mango offers vitamins and natural sweetness. This pudding supports gut health and satisfies sweet cravings.

Preparation Time: 15 minutes (plus chilling time)

7. Turmeric Roasted Nuts:

Ingredients:

- ✓ 1 cup mixed nuts (almonds, walnuts, cashews)
- ✓ 1 tablespoon olive oil
- ✓ 1 teaspoon ground turmeric
- ✓ 1/2 teaspoon ground cumin
- ✓ 1/2 teaspoon smoked paprika
- ✓ Salt to taste

Instructions:

- ✓ Preheat the oven to 350°F (175°C).
- ✓ In a bowl, toss mixed nuts with olive oil, turmeric, cumin, smoked paprika, and salt.
- ✓ Spread the nuts on a baking sheet in a single layer.
- ✓ Roast in the oven for 12-15 minutes, stirring halfway through.
- ✓ Allow to cool before serving.

Health Benefits:

- ✓ Nuts offer healthy fats and protein, while turmeric provides anti-inflammatory properties. This savory snack supports gut health and provides a satisfying and flavorful option.

Preparation Time: 20 minutes

8. Probiotic Yogurt Parfait with Berries:

Ingredients:

- ✓ 1 cup plain Greek yogurt (unsweetened)
- ✓ 1/2 cup mixed berries (blueberries, strawberries)
- ✓ 2 tablespoons granola (low in added sugars)
- ✓ 1 tablespoon honey or maple syrup
- ✓ 1 tablespoon flaxseeds (ground)

Instructions:

- ✓ In a glass or bowl, layer plain Greek yogurt at the bottom.
- ✓ Add a layer of mixed berries.
- ✓ Sprinkle granola and ground flaxseeds over the berries.
- ✓ Drizzle honey or maple syrup on top.
- ✓ Repeat for additional layers.
- ✓ Serve chilled.

Health Benefits:

- ✓ This probiotic-rich parfait supports gut health with Greek yogurt, while berries and flaxseeds contribute fiber and antioxidants. It's a delicious and nutritious snack option.

Preparation Time: 5 minutes

9. Veggie and Hummus Stuffed Avocado:

Ingredients:

- ✓ 2 avocados, halved and pitted
- ✓ 1/2 cup hummus (homemade or store-bought)
- ✓ Assorted veggies for stuffing (cherry tomatoes, cucumber, bell peppers)
- ✓ Sprouts or microgreens for garnish
- ✓ Lemon wedges for serving

Instructions:

- ✓ Scoop out a small portion of the avocado to create a well.
- ✓ Fill each avocado half with hummus.
- ✓ Stuff with assorted veggies of your choice.
- ✓ Garnish with sprouts or microgreens.
- ✓ Serve with lemon wedges for squeezing.

Health Benefits:

- ✓ Avocado provides healthy fats, hummus offers plant-based protein, and the assortment of veggies contributes fiber and essential nutrients, promoting gut health.

Preparation Time: 10 minutes

10. Beetroot and Goat Cheese Dip:

Ingredients:

- ✓ 1 cup roasted beetroot, diced
- ✓ 1/2 cup goat cheese
- ✓ 2 tablespoons Greek yogurt (unsweetened)
- ✓ 1 tablespoon olive oil
- ✓ 1 clove garlic, minced
- ✓ Salt and pepper to taste
- ✓ Whole grain crackers or vegetable sticks for dipping

Instructions:

- ✓ In a food processor, blend roasted beetroot, goat cheese, Greek yogurt, olive oil, and minced garlic until smooth.
- ✓ Season with salt and pepper to taste.
- ✓ Transfer the dip to a serving bowl.
- ✓ Serve with whole grain crackers or vegetable sticks for dipping.

Health Benefits:

- ✓ This vibrant dip combines the antioxidants from beetroots with probiotics from Greek yogurt and the creamy texture of goat cheese, offering a flavorful and gut-friendly snack.

Preparation Time: 15 minutes

CONCLUSION

This gut health cookbook serves as a comprehensive guide to cultivating a vibrant and balanced digestive system through the art of mindful and nourishing cooking.

We've explored a diverse array of recipes designed not only to tantalize your taste buds but also to promote a flourishing gut microbiome. By incorporating probiotic-rich foods, fiber-packed ingredients, and anti-inflammatory spices, these recipes aim to support digestive wellness and overall health.

Our culinary journey has highlighted the interconnectedness of good nutrition and gut health, emphasizing the significance of fostering a diverse and harmonious microbiota.

From breakfast bowls bursting with antioxidants to savory lunches loaded with fiber, and wholesome snacks that nurture your gut flora, these recipes are crafted with a thoughtful blend of flavors and nutritional benefits.

As you embark on this gastronomic adventure, consider this cookbook not just as a collection of recipes but as a holistic approach to well-being. May the flavors and nourishment found within these pages inspire you to embark on a lifelong journey of culinary exploration, where each meal becomes an opportunity to enhance not only your taste experience but also the health and vitality of your gut. Cheers to a happy and healthy digestive journey!